CW00518261

DEDICATION

I dedicate my first book to my amazing father John Coley. His constant encouragement and praise has empowered me to consistently be the best version of me.

I also dedicate it to You the reader and promoter of your own health.

Orgasmic Health

Annie Day

ORGASMIC HEALTH

Copyright

Copyright © 2018 ANNIE DAY

First Printing: 2018

ISBN-10: 1983705772

ISBN-13: 978-1983705779

ANNIE DAY

UNITED KINGDOM

www.heavenscentbliss.co.uk

CONTENTS

ACKNOWLEDGEMENTS

Thank you to all my Soul Sisters and Brothers for your Love, Support and Honesty in giving me your authentic feedback on my first book *Orgasmic Health*. I am also grateful for you reminding me how wonderfully gifted I am. Thank you from the bottom of my heart. I feel blessed beyond measure that you honour me with your friendship.

I wish to thank all of the website owners who have kindly given permission to cite their pages and to Iona light who has also kindly donated their water cleanse illustration.

Disclaimer

This book is not intended to be a substitute for medical advice or treatment. Any person with a condition requiring medical advice or attention should consult with a qualified medical practitioner.

INTRODUCTION

Annie Day MSc. Cert Med Ed.

I'm Annie Day, owner of Heaven Scent Bliss, I use my many years of experience and comprehensive knowledge to help you to reach optimum health, surpass your goals and to consistently be the best version of yourself.

Our Mission

Our mission is to be a quality provider of a comprehensive range of complementary therapies and to be a learning provider of distinction.

To meet a diverse range of Mind, Body and Spiritual needs for all clients who find their way to us.

You will get unique, individual treatments in a serene and relaxed environment, with a friendly and caring approach by Annie herself.

Enjoy reading my book, if you want to find out more take a look at my website www.heavenscentbliss.co.uk or contact me at annie@heavenscentbliss.co.uk.

I guarantee that if you have a treatment with me you will experience **Heaven Scent Bliss**

With Love & Blessings Annie x x

1

Water

Our bodies are composed of over 70% water so it is important that we are replacing water lost through respiration, urination, digestion and perspiration, with good quality water. A visual reminder is if you consider your body to be a Ferrari – a real supercharged, gorgeous, high-energy vehicle – would you really put inferior fuel inside it? Of course not. We know that if we put inferior fuel into our Ferrari it would be unable to provide optimum energy and this would have a negative effect on its performance and longevity.

I have read some interesting articles regarding tap water which suggest that tap water contains: chlorine, fluoride, pesticides, insecticides, herbicides, heavy metals, female hormones and everyone else's medication. This revelation made me rethink drinking tap water, and as a result I wanted to explore other ways to keep hydrated, especially as I had recently been suffering with low energy. As a result, a naturopathic doctor advised me to stop drinking tap water, as he felt it was having such a negative effect on me.

It is alleged there are many issues with fluoride too. Although, where it occurs naturally with other trace elements means it is good for dental health. However, I believe the man-made variety has a negative impact as it contains a neurotoxin. There are some interesting articles out there for you to research, if you care to look, and make informed choices on what is the best way forward for yourself. Take a look at the health nuts news website which has some great tips and articles for you to peruse at your leisure: www.healthnutnews.com.

Having done research for my personal and professional benefit, not least because I have a low tolerance to tap water; for the last two years I've been drinking Kangen water, which is provided through a Japanese medical device system. Basically, it's a machine with filters in it that removes all of the toxins and medication from tap water. This machine also alkalises the water, with one of the benefits being that the molecules become smaller so that our bodies, at a cellular level, are better hydrated. It is quite simply antioxidant alkaline water; this water is said to help boost your immune system, improve your circulation, maximise your digestive processes, detoxifying your whole system and even reverse the signs of ageing. There are numerous YouTube videos that demonstrate the benefits of drinking alkalised water.

From my personal perspective, I love the way I feel drinking this life-giving water and have a similar system called an Anespa, which takes out harmful chlorine and fluoride from my bath and shower water. This means I am literally bathing in beautiful mineral water. The benefits I first discovered were that my skin was even softer, and that I no longer felt itchy after a shower, as I previously did using tap water. If you live local to me then please do come and take a bottle of Kangen water to trial. If you'd like to do a three-week trial to see the amazing benefits, then simply contact me via email annie@heavenscentbliss.co.uk.

I also believe there are benefits to eating alkalised food. I have read articles which suggest that cancer cannot survive in an alkaline system, along with many other conditions including: chronic fatigue syndrome, arthritis and auto immune diseases.

Having looked at the quality of the water there are other factors that determine how much benefit we can get from our water. For instance, by drinking warm room temperature water our bodies and digestive system can more easily assimilate warm water as it is already at body temperature. By drinking cold water, especially refrigerated water, it can take up to two hours for your body to get it to the right temperature for usage. I am infamous for turning up at networking and social events with my own flask of Kangen water, with half hot and half cold water in it so that I can remain healthy throughout the day. Sometimes the timing of drinking water is critical too; for instance, by drinking water half an hour before eating food can enhance how effectively our bodies are able to assimilate and digest the food we have eaten.

Many of us take water up to bed with us. While this is a good practice, it can also help with hydration, especially if you wake up during the night to urinate. It is ultra-important that you protect your drinking water by covering it up whilst you are asleep at night. There are many reasons for doing this: 1) you may find that there are toxins in the air that find their way into your glass and 2) we release lots of negativity whilst we are sleeping, so this can also be present in your water. So, simply place a coaster or a sheet of card over it until you are ready to drink it. Should you wake up during the night you can sip from it and cover it up again in the sure knowledge that you are drinking good quality water that will enhance your body's health.

Iona light offer a water cleanse mat, see next page, or go to www.Iona-light.co.uk for more information.

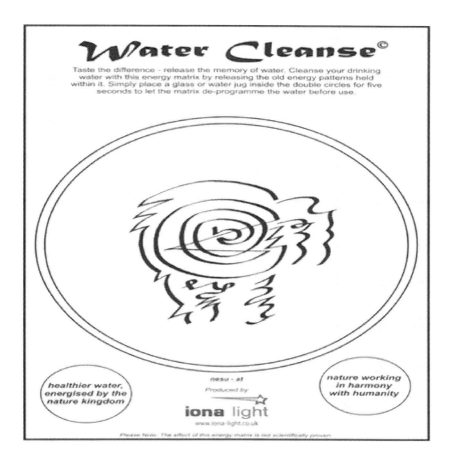

Bathing and Showering. As well as water having an impact on us through drinking and cooking, I believe we should address the issue of bathing and showering in tap water too. Anything that we place on our skin from skin creams, essential oils, shampoo and water, takes less than 4 minutes before it is absorbed by our major organs, especially the liver. There are healthy options available, namely Kangen water, which is the equivalent of bathing in mineral water and has no chlorine in it. Another option is Reverse Osmosis which also takes chlorine out; however, it is in effect 'dead water' as it contains no minerals at all and is still acidic water which is considered less healthy for humans than alkalised water. There are companies on the internet that sell effective de-chlorinators for the shower and bath. These are an economical solution, especially for sufferers of eczema and those who are sensitive to chlorine and fluoride, particularly children.

Another positive strategy when using water is to talk positively to it. Thanks to the work of Masaru Emoto who basically freezes water that has been spoken to kindly, then, before it can defrost completely, he takes photos of it. This water produces the most beautiful snowflake patterns. He did likewise with water that had been told that it was ugly and bad and this water when photographed produced deformed patterns. I fully recommend the book *Hidden Messages in Water*, which introduces the revolutionary work of internationally renowned Japanese scientist Masaru Emoto. He discovered that molecules in water are affected by our thoughts, words and feelings.

The strategy I recommended is to get a glass bottle that is at least 1.5 litres, this is so you have an accurate measurement of how much good quality water you are drinking daily, especially whilst you are at work. It is sometimes difficult to judge how many glasses of water you've had throughout the day so by using the standard 1.5 litres you have a measurement, whereby you can add more if necessary. I would recommend drinking water from a glass bottle, rather than a plastic bottle; with plastic bottles there is the danger that phyto-oestrogens will bleed into your water. Phyto-oestrogens are well known carcinogens.

Here are some of the conditions that have been shown through research to benefit from a balanced increase of water:

Angina - water shortage in the heart and lung axis

Arthritis - dehydration in the joint cavities

Asthma - drought management programmes in the body

Autoimmune diseases

Back pain - water shortages in the spinal column and discs

Colitis - water shortage in the large gut

Diabetes - some cells getting only survival rations of water

Heartburn - water shortage in the upper gastrointestinal tract

High blood cholesterol - early drought management by the body

High blood pressure - lack of water to fill blood vessels that defuse water into vital cells

Migraines - water shortage in the brain and eyes

Pain - the body is unable to release the pain from muscular aches and pains.

Some easy tips for drinking more water are:

Start the day with a glass of warm water.

Keep a glass of water near you and sip it often throughout the day.

When you feel thirsty, drink water first rather than any other liquid.

When you are hungry drink water first and if you still feel hungry a short time later eat some sensible food.

Every time you have a stimulant such as tea, coffee or alcohol, follow it with a glass of water, preferably warm.

Experiment with drinking warm water instead of tea or coffee.

2

Sleep

One of the benefits of a good night sleep is that the body can restore and repair. When we are sleep deprived it can have a negative impact on our mind, body and spirit. That is why during the Second World War this was used as a form of torture, as sleep deprivation has such a devastating effect upon us.

How much do you need? It varies for each individual, and as a rough guide eight hours is the optimum amount for most of us. Many things can have an impact on our sleep quality and duration, not least chronic and acute stress. Also, eating late in the evening can have an impact on how easily we sleep. A good rule of thumb is to eat no later than 8pm if you are going to sleep at 11pm. This is because it takes approximately three hours for your body to digest food. Any food which has not been processed within that three hours will turn to sugar, which can be disruptive for our blood sugar levels and put an additional strain on the digestive organs, especially the liver. In Chinese medicine we believe that there is a system called the Horary Cycle, which shows at what point of the day your body and specific organs are working at their optimum effectiveness.

So, for instance, if you are waking up consistently between 3am and 5am it could be because your lung and liver meridian is working especially hard to process things on your behalf. The liver is said to represent fear, irritation, disappointment and anger, whilst the lungs are concerned with unresolved loss and grief issues. Sometimes just knowing why you are waking up can be helpful in determining what support you may need to resolve these issues.

Something I teach my patients who have suffered, or who are suffering from chronic insomnia, is how to sedate the adrenal glands using hand reflexology. Basically, starting at the middle outside edge of your thumb, using the index finger from your other hand, slide diagonally across to the centre of the palm of your hand. This is where your adrenal glands are situated just above the kidneys. So, with that index finger do gentle circular motions massaging gently away from the thumb. Then do the same on the other hand. This is best done just before you retire, should you wake up during the night simply do it again. This will get your body back into a positive pattern and will promote restful sleep for you.

Additionally, watching and listening to the news throughout the day and especially in the evening can mean that painful, negative and challenging images are still playing on your mind as the negative words are embedded. Many of us who have been sensitive to the news in the past and acknowledge that our insomnia was caused by this issue choose to watch less, or to stop watching earlier in the evening. Many years ago, a therapist challenged me to stop engaging with the news in any format for three weeks. I accepted the challenge and discovered that I was far more peaceful and slept restfully as a result. The news can increase stress levels and heighten our fight or flight response.

I believe that the adage 'No News is Good News' applies very well here. Although it usually applies to a situation for instance, when a loved one is in hospital and we believe that the fact that the hospital hasn't phoned us means its good news. There is a monthly newspaper called Good News that is available from www.goodnewsnetwork.org, it carries lots of wonderful articles about the heroism in the world, and the beautiful kind and loving experiences that are happening globally.

How much water should you drink before bed? A good strategy is to stop drinking tea or coffee at 6pm so that you are only drinking good quality water for the rest of the evening, thus hydrating the body.

Several strategies that may promote restful sleep include listening to music, lighting a candle or having a warm bath before bed. Write down ten things before you sleep that you are grateful for during the day. For five minutes before retiring, lie on your back, with your legs raised high up as this can help your heart to rest. Ensure that within the bedroom environment there are as few electrical devices as possible. If you do have a TV in your bedroom unplug it at night, because if you leave it on standby I believe it is emitting an electromagnetic field (EMF) which can be agitating and cause anxiety during your sleep time. If you must use your phone as an alarm you can fix it with a resonator available from www.quantumk.co.uk.

If you have absorbed EMFs you may find that your legs are twitching whilst you're in bed, which is sometimes referred to as 'restless legs'. You may find that you feel agitated and angry for no apparent reason. Other symptoms may include feeling exhausted and out of sorts, where there is no rhyme or reason for you to be feeling like this. All you need to address this is a domestic hairdryer; it can be as economical as you like. The procedure that you're going to use is called degaussing. The most important part of the hairdryer is the motor at the back of the hairdryer, as within motor there are magnets that are spinning. When you are experiencing some or all of the symptoms mentioned above, simply plug in the hairdryer (if you have long hair like myself, tie it up). Turn the hairdryer on, use any heat setting that you prefer then run the back of the hairdryer around your aura as close to your physical body as possible. I generally do this two or three times; ensure that you don't get the motor too close to you. When you've done that take the motor of the hairdryer (the back of it) and while it is still plugged in and working take the hairdryer from your crown all the way down to your feet. The magnets in effect break up the EMF field. This has instantaneous benefits and usually helps you to feel positive, lighter and more optimistic. The next time you're experiencing some of the symptoms associated with EMFs just give the degaussing procedure a whirl.

3

Food

For many years I have practised as a kinesiologist and nutritionist, and whenever I do an allergy test the foods that are the most problematic for many us are genetically modified organisms: GMO. Our bodies accurately recognise them as 'alien', as they are not natural foods from our planet. For example, I have a low tolerance to Monosodium glutamate: abbreviated to (MSG).

Whenever my friends invite me to go out for a Chinese meal or Thai meal we ask if they can guarantee that there will be no MSG in any of my food. We have usually explained that in the past I have experienced anaphylactic shock from eating food that was supposed to not have MSG in it. My patients tell me it is sometimes worth explaining how sensitive we are so that the members of staff are not tempted to put just a tiny bit in. Another food that is said to harm people is Aspartame, which is another genetically modified organism that is highly addictive. It is typically found in diet drinks, carbonated drinks, squashes, fruit juices, yoghurts and desserts.

The history of GMO wheat began many years ago when the Russians decided that they would genetically modify their wheat so that it had a higher yield. The Russians then sold it to the Americans who decided that they wanted this GM wheat to grow lower on the stalk so that it would be possible to have smaller combine harvesters. Some years later the Americans then sold this to the Canadians; where the Canadians decided that they wanted to add a pesticide to this GM wheat that grew lower on the stalk and had a higher yield. It is predominantly Canadian wheat that is in the majority of wheat flour in the UK, which is a huge problem for many people, especially those suffering from chronic fatigue syndrome (CFS), coeliac's and those who are sensitive to GMOs and glycophosphates.

I discovered some years ago that whenever I travelled to France to stay with friends who lived there, that my body could tolerate lots of lovely French bread and French pastries with no side effects at all. When I spoke to my friends about this anomaly, as they are ex-farmers, they explained that in France French farmers believe that their wheat is wonderful exactly as it is.

There is a variety of foods which are organic, free range and with the creatures' best interests at heart. We've known for many years that we are what we eat and what we can absorb, so it is best to ensure that most of the food that we are eating is organic.

Over the last seven years there has been a really big increase in the amount of rapeseed that has been grown in the UK. This was said to be since the EU began subsidising farmers to grow this crop. However, I have noticed there has been a huge increase in the amount of people who are affected negatively by rapeseed pollen, especially children, the elderly and infirm who are coming for allergy testing appointments. The main foods which have rapeseed in them are: mayonnaise, salad cream, humus, guacamole, ready prepared coleslaw and potato salad.

Why not try the organic box system; there are many different companies available, depending on the area of the country that you are living in. Typically, they offer a fruit and veg box for a small, medium-sized or large family. It is usually possible to select only fruits and vegetables that you and your family enjoy and there is normally an option for you to select your favourites. The beauty of this is that the produce comes only from the UK, it is grown locally and therefore has no air miles attached, which is a healthy and economical way of buying good quality organic fruit and veg. Some companies also sell organic fish, meat and dairy products. It's worth shopping around to find the company that would deliver to you, with the options that are most important to you and your family.

Food combinations are based on the work of the Hayes Diet, where fruit is eaten first thing in the morning on its own and a gap of an hour is left before either protein or carbohydrate is eaten. The theory behind this is that the fructose present in the fruit will be processed quickly in the body, so it needs to be digested separately to any other food substance. The rest of the meals within the food combining template are meals that will either be protein plus salad or vegetables, or carbohydrates with salad or vegetables. For example, when using the food combining style of eating, it would be possible to have as a carbohydrate meal: a jacket potato with butter, humus and salad, as these are all carbohydrate rich foods. It would not be possible to add to the jacket potato tuna, beans or cheese as these are all proteins. The way that we process carbohydrates and proteins and the speed at which this varies is significant, hence this method which keeps proteins and carbohydrates separate. This often means that the person loses weight, even though this is not a diet as such, simply a healthy way of eating that is kind on the digestive system.

Eating right for your blood type is another style of eating that can be beneficial. It is one that I've adopted over the last couple of years and which has kept my weight and blood sugar levels stable; there are books available about this.

My blood type is O negative, so for me wheat is one of the foods that my body would find most difficult to process. Dairy is also challenging for my digestive system to process, whereas walnuts, pumpkin seeds, sunflower seeds, fish of all kinds and organic chicken are all easy for an O negative body to assimilate and absorb the nutrients from. Fortunately, the foods that are on the NO list of foods I don't generally enjoy, whereas the foods on the YES list are typically foods that I really enjoy. I have discovered that many of my patient's family and friends who have engaged with this notion of eating right for your blood type have really benefited from this system.

There are many benefits to eating raw food and juicing.

Many people have seen significant weight loss, huge increases in energy and vitality, which helps them to be motivated to do exercise, engage in races and to take up more lively activities. By eating raw food, none of the natural occurring vitamins, minerals and Omegas is reduced by cooking and refining, thus the individual gains the optimum amount of energy from each bit of food digested. Many people are adding juicing to their breakfast and daily healthy routine. There are many juicing machines on the market. By doing a little research you will be able to find the one that is most appropriate for you and that fits in with your budget and the amount of time you've got to juice.

Another strategy to balance blood sugar and stabilise one's weight is to eat a low GI diet. The principle behind this way of eating is to maintain energy throughout the day. With this theory it is said to be important to eat little and often, to ensure blood sugar levels remain stable. It is vital to eat foods that release sugar into the blood slowly; these are called low glycaemic foods. If you also need to control your weight it is advisable to keep your saturated fats to a minimum, but do ensure that you are getting plenty of good fats. The general principle is to eat small frequent meals, preferably containing some proteins. In this system it is said to be imperative that the person eats breakfast, avoids sugar and sugar containing foods; fruit juices should be avoided and dried fruit intake kept to a minimum.

People using this system are encouraged to avoid alcohol, reduce caffeine and are encouraged to take regular exercise daily. Without going into too many details the basic premise is that you eat well at breakfast and have a drink of either hot water with lemon or weak Indian or herbal tea, at mid-morning a drink of your choice, plus a snack. Next you have lunch, which will consist of meat, fish, eggs, poultry or pulses with a large salad. Again, you have a snack and a drink around mid-afternoon. Dinner consists of a serving of fish, turkey or chicken with at least three vegetables, brown or wild rice or noodles as an example. Then there will be a drink and a bedtime snack. Some of the foods which have the lowest GI are: pulses, cherries, onions, broad beans, barley, avocados, mushrooms, sprouts, apples, courgettes, leafy greens, mangetout, apricots, spinach, leeks, yoghurt, grapefruit, peppers, green beans and peanuts.

Medium GI foods include: sweet potatoes, raw carrots, whole wheat pasta, oats, buckwheat, grapes, mangoes, sweetcorn, noodles, oranges, beetroot, yams, peas, figs, wholegrain breads, Basmati and brown rice, kiwi fruits and fresh dates.

High GI foods are: glucose, pineapple, watermelon, parsnips, swede, rice cakes, cornflakes, sugar, bananas, baked potatoes, cooked carrots, rye crisp breads, couscous, instant oats cereal, honey, raisins, mashed potatoes, squash, white bread and breadsticks.

Foods that are said to heal, means consuming more whole foods including at least five portions of fruit and vegetables, nuts and seeds with adequate essential fatty acids, proteins and drinking plenty of water. Eat slow releasing carbohydrates, fruit, vegetables and all oily fish. Use snacks to balance blood sugar levels, for example oatcakes, nuts, seeds and fruit. By ensuring that your blood sugar levels are balanced there is less chance that low blood sugar levels will force you into eating junk food, which is essentially unhealthy for you.

4

Exercise

We have been told for years that we need to do plenty of exercise; no pain no gain is the way we should be looking at our exercise strategies.

If the above practice isn't your cup of tea try power walking for ten minutes twice daily. Stand up as much as possible. If your career involves lots of sitting down have yourself tested for an ergonomic seat and check your desk position. This can make all the difference to your spinal health. Experiment with dance classes; again, make sure it's something that you enjoy. There is plenty available depending on the area that you live in so give Zumba, Ceroc, Salsa, Belly Dancing and Dancercise – this is where you dance holding glow in the dark sticks – a go. One of my personal favourites is rebounding, which I tend to do for ten minutes morning and evening. It may be that you enjoy weight training, if this is the case make sure that you go to a gym and have a proper safety induction, so you do not overstretch your body and injure it. If you'd like to take up running find a local group to go with, as often, when we do things in groups, we are much better motivated to turn up consistently. For those of you who can tolerate chlorine the local pool might be a good way of you doing exercise, including everything from doing lengths to aqua aerobics.

Take the stairs not the lift. Have a brisk walk daily. Even ten minutes can make an enormous difference to your mood and give you vital sunlight that can activate vitamin D3.

Allow yourself time for recovery and rest. Start your day with simple exercises every morning using stretching, toning and warm up movements. Additionally, gentle Tai Chi movements can be a good way of loosening up your body, help with your breathing and reduce stress levels. If you enjoy yoga that can also be a good way of giving your body positive energy and can also reduce stress levels. For times when you know that you want to do a lot of exercise, for example because you are taking part in a race of some kind or you are a triathlete, the benefits of regular chiropractor treatments can ensure that you soon recover from any injuries quickly and can protect your body from further injury. As a kinesiologist I often help triathletes manage their diets, exercise programs, training and rest periods, so that they are able to continue to beat their personal best. It can make a significant difference to performance levels and reduce injuries. Most importantly, find a therapist that is recommended and that you trust to help you get the most from your diet and your exercise programme. Enjoy it. Exercise is so good for our hearts, so ensure that you're enjoying exercise that you love.

*Remember to visit your GP first if you have any ongoing illnesses or have not exercised in a long time to make sure it is safe to do so.

5

Healthy Mind and Body

Essential oils can be excellent for a whole range of issues as they heal our body, mind and soul. One of my favourites is Frankincense as its psychological benefit is that it helps us to let go on every level, it releases fears from the past and promotes hope for the future. Letting go of the past is an important strategy so that we can move on. Often when people are feeling sad it is because they are not engaging in the present moment, they are still thinking about things from the past. However bad the past was it has made you the amazing person that you are today. Once we have made our peace with the past we can enjoy the present moment and move forward into a bright future. If you're finding it difficult to do this then find a therapist that you trust to explore this with so that you can have the life that you want and deserve.

Here are my favourite essential oils. Rosemary is a memory booster and antidepressant. Tea tree is anti-viral, antifungal, anti-septic and antibiotic, whilst also stimulating the immunity system. Geranium is a good balancer of our hormones as well as our emotions, plus I love the fragrance of it. I use Litsea cubeba (may chang) to fragrance my bathroom as it smells very citrusy and fresh. For a stimulating warming bath, I run my bath to the right height and temperature and then add two drops of ginger. By using only a small amount of essential oils, we are doing what is called 'subtle aromatherapy'. By using less essential oil it has an impact on the body, mind and spirit; whereas, when we use lots of aromatherapy oils it will only work on our physicality. When using aromatherapy oils remember that less is more. Why don't you pick up a book on the benefits of aromatherapy oils to get you started? Or try the Aromatherapy Lexicon, which is easy to use as a great reference guide for a comprehensive range of conditions.

Most books will concentrate on the physical aspects, so what could be more useful to you is if I gave you the psychological aspects of essential oils:

Basil for concentration and understanding

Benzoin for self-love and clarity

Bergamot for acceptance and honesty

Black Pepper for excitement

Grapefruit for certainty and trust

Fennel for hope and peace

Frankincense for letting go

Geranium for balance and flexibility

Ginger for forbearance

Jasmine for ecstasy and exhilaration

Lavender for insight

Lemon for change and influence

Mandarin for childhood and happiness

Marjoram for the frequency of order

Patchouli for wants and desires

Sweet Orange for joy and happiness

Rosemary for learning and self-will

Sandalwood for protection and confidence

Tea Tree for cleanliness and purity

And finally, Ylang Ylang for truth and nerve.

One of the most important things that we can do for ourselves is to ensure that we have daily opportunities for relaxation. This could include having an aromatherapy massage or reflexology for instance, as these can help to release stress and anxiety. It is vital that we maintain a balance between work, rest and play for our overall well-being. We tend to be applauded for continual overwork, and to be praised for working long hours, skipping meals and having very little time for recreation and time with our families. If we could just look at ourselves holistically we would gain a better understanding of how important rest, fun and pleasure are. Today treat yourself as if you were your own best friend. Give this *'friend'* lots of compliments about how well they are doing. Affirm yourself. I guarantee this will be beneficial when you do this consistently.

Make sure that this *'friend'* finishes work on time and sets aside some relaxation and fun time. By making this commitment to yourself you are setting up a good habit. One of the strategies I suggest to my patients is to write down a relaxing treat, pamper treatment or a nature walk in your diary for twenty-one days. It is said in many cultures and by many psychologists that any habit that you do for twenty-one days becomes an ingrained behaviour. So, whilst we may have less healthy addictions such as drinking or smoking, that have a negative impact on us, the 'make time for me' daily strategy can have a significant positive impact.

I cannot stress enough the importance of daily affirmations for fulfilling daily experiences. Start each day with gratitude for at least ten things. I began using my daily affirmations so that I have the best possible outcomes for each day. One of the ways that I lock in these affirmations is to use a technique called Havening. This technique involves self-touch, stroking slowly both hands from the shoulders to the wrist, then stroking the palms across each other, finally stroking from the forehead down the sides of the face. Use this technique to manifest and visualise your dreams becoming a reality.

Here are the affirmations that my patients, and myself, use most frequently:

I am a magnet for prosperity and abundance.

Everything I touch is successful.

Everything I touch turns to gold.

I am a brilliant manifester and I'm already manifesting great health and energy.

The law of attraction brings only good into my life.

Life supports me in every way.

I lovingly do everything I can to assist my body in maintaining perfect health.

I get plenty of sleep every night and my body appreciates it.

I deserve the best and now I accept the best.

I balance my life between work, rest and play, so they all get equal time.

Ideas come to me easily and effortlessly.

My life gets more fabulous every day. I look forward to what each new hour brings.

I am a radiant being enjoying life to the fullest.

Right now, enormous wealth and power are available to me. I choose to be worthy and deserving.

My job allows me to express my talents and abilities, and I'm grateful for this employment.

My wealth comes from expected and unexpected sources.

My unique talents and abilities are always in great demand.

I am grateful for being alive today. It is my joy and pleasure to live another wonderful day.

I have the perfect relationship now.

I have a happy, sexual, spiritual relationship now with someone who loves and respects me.

I am happy standing in my feminine/masculine power.

Thank you for all I have. All I've had. And all I will have.

It does not matter what others say or do. All that matters is how I choose to react and what I choose to believe about myself.

All is well in my world and all is in divine and perfect order.

Right now, I have a brilliant...memory, body, confidence, job, relationship etc.

We often limit ourselves by believing that we are not worthy of the amazing blessings that the universe has to offer. A way around this is to imagine that the universe is the best parent ever in the world. This parent wants to spoil you with all the gifts that could possibly help you physically, emotionally and psychologically. Especially when working with children I ask them to imagine that the universe is a Genie who can grant any wish that you can think of, providing you think you deserve it. So, one of the affirmations that is quite useful for this is the – I deserve and accept the best that the universe can offer. A great gratitude one is: thank you for all I have, all I have had and all I will have. Reach for the stars and think big!

One of the best gifts we can give ourselves is self-forgiveness and loving ourselves unconditionally. Often, we are very good at doing this for other people and not so good at doing it for ourselves. As soon as we start to love ourselves unconditionally we attract other people who love and respect us, and we start to receive huge gifts in the way of ideas, increasing finances and unexpected windfalls of blessings.

6

EMFs – Electro Magnetic Fields

Electricity is a godsend for many reasons, from the common electric light to powering up hospitals, schools, restaurants, hotels etc. However, it does have a negative impact on us as well, as it means that we can work from dawn until dusk once daylight has disappeared. If you find that you are being affected adversely, you can buy beautiful pendants and other jewellery that protect you from EMFs and Wi-Fi. Another valuable resource is Quantum K resonators available from www.quantumk.com. These are small copper rectangles that have been programmed to protect you and which can be applied to all electrical devices.

For people that are wary of having mammograms, there is a more natural and non-invasive process which doesn't use radiation, it is a system called medical thermography. This system looks at your temperature throughout your body and shows areas of heat, which could mean that there is a problem in that area. You can read more about it on the internet.

There are usually clinics set up all over the UK where staff members bring the machines to a local venue, whereby appointments are set up prior to this. It is pain free, natural and an effective way of looking at your body: detecting any anomalies early so that interventions can be taken if necessary. I personally have found the imaging to be relaxing and effective.

7

Avoiding Stress

To ensure that you are as positive and as happy as possible it is important to avoid, as much as possible, negative situations, places and people. Irrespective of whether you believe in angels or not, Archangel Michael is a protective Angel, so as soon as you become conscious of a negative situation call him in. It doesn't need to be elaborate, simply say Archangel Michael protect me. Imagine putting on colourful sparkling armour that only allows 100% love and positivity in. Additionally, imagine Teflon coating your aura in your favourite colour.

Again, define your intention so that your Teflon coated aura will only allow 100% love and positivity in. We fully appreciate that we live in an amazing, beautiful, fantastic world and also acknowledge the Yin Yang principle. The balance of life means we have to experience good as well as bad, without night there would be no day. We need the polarities so that we can experience the beautiful and the profound. So, by acknowledging that we need protection we are simply giving ourselves the opportunity to shine like the superstars we are; by being a shining light that is not manipulated or dimmed by lower energies.

The most difficult places are clearly the most negative, especially for sensitive people and empathic folk. I find that the most notorious places for negative energy are airports, supermarkets, theatres and large public venues. If you know you are going to be in places like this there is a need to additionally protect yourself so that you are not adversely affected by the negativity and lower energies of the place.

Many of us experience feeling very tired after we have spent time with negative people. These people are often needy and simply love high vibrational energy, and people who are joyful and happy. They become 'energy vampires' as they take our energy and attempt to feel better. By protecting ourselves, as described earlier, we can be kind, loving and empathic, and not allow this energy vampirism to affect us unduly. Just ten minutes of walking in nature can reset our energy and help us feel more grounded and at peace. By simply looking at so much greenery, it can calm us and help us to put our lives in perspective. The trees can teach us much about grounding, as they have as much roots below the ground as they have branches above the ground.

It is excellent that we allow ourselves to engage with spiritual activities, and it is also especially important that we ground ourselves so that we can do the spiritual work that we came here to do, so that we can manifest our dreams into reality.

8

Beauty and Personal Care Products

There are many concerns about using some skin care products, such as shampoos, deodorants, toothpaste, lotions and toners, which contain parabens. These are present in a lot of commercially produced products. The companies that do not use parabens, SLS and phylates, proclaim it loud and proud on their packaging. Another additive is Sodium Lauryl Sulphate (SLS) and Sodium Laureth Sulphate (SLES), which is generally found in deodorants, toothpaste and shampoo.

To get your home and work smelling wonderful why not try using essential oils, substituting these for cleaning products. I make a great oven cleaner that is composed of Cornish sea salt, essential oils of sweet orange, lime, grapefruit, May Chang and lemongrass. I apply it to the oven, leave it for a couple of hours, then give it a scrub and with very little effort it is shiny, sparkly and smells great. I use vinegar to clean windows and shower doors adding a couple of drops of sweet orange essential oil to fragrance the bathroom.

There are a lot of organic cleaning products available; it is worth shopping around to see which you like best.

9

How Quickly We Get Results from a Healthy Lifestyle

It is essential to let go of addictions as soon as possible, whilst also being kind and loving to yourself as you go through this positive process. Although nicotine has had lots of bad press in the past, the current trend of using vaping also has acute drawbacks; current research suggests that it can cause an incurable lung disease called "popcorn lung". This is worrying as many young people especially, erroneously believe that it is a safe alternative to smoking nicotine as a cigarette. As vaping is a fairly new concept there have been no opportunities to do a longitudinal study over a significant period of time which would provide valuable information on the consequences of using this system.

There are various strategies that you can use to give up smoking and drinking alcohol. Some of the tried and tested and effective routes seem to be: acupuncture, hypnosis, hypnotherapy, visualisations, aromatherapy oils and having a goal, so that each pound that you would have spent you put towards, for instance, a holiday or a new car. By using any or all of these methods, means that you can make a significant and positive difference to your life and increase your own lifespan too.

For those who drink every day the most significant change you could make would be to reduce your alcohol consumption, as alcohol interferes with your sleep pattern. It prevents you from having rapid eye movement's, sometimes referred to as REM. For you to have a restful sleep you need to go into the stage of REM so that you can go into a deeper sleep. As alcohol disrupts this, it means that you are not dreaming, which is an important healing and restorative mechanism for the body, mind and spirit. So, start by having one less drink per week or perhaps having a drink of water after each alcoholic drink.

The guidance of a therapist can help you overcome this addiction. Remember any steps that you make, however small, are taking you towards your end goal. We often treat ourselves badly when we are overcoming addiction and beat ourselves up when we fall off the wagon, so to speak. If you do hit a glitch, simply start again and remember that you can only do your best. Enjoy the health benefits that you receive as a bonus for overcoming your addiction. We are all a work in progress, so enjoy the journey.

10

Environment and Sustainability

Although this is a relatively small chapter it was still an important statement to make. By taking care of our beautiful blue-green planet, we are actually taking care of ourselves as well. By eating organic and free-range products that are grown in the UK, we are supporting the economy as well as our health. We are not incurring air miles by insisting on having products that would not be available usually and naturally, for example strawberries in November. We are being encouraged to do more for recycling than any other time in our history, which must clearly have an impact on our planet and is a way of giving our children and grandchildren a healthy legacy for the future.

By finding environmentally friendly solutions for energy, such as wind turbines and wave power, means that we will not be so dependent upon fossil fuels, and as a result will be leaving less of a carbon footprint. As our technologies improve we may find other natural, planet friendly solutions that are sustainable as food sources, energy sources and for accommodating all of the inhabitants of Earth.

11

Orgasmic Sex

As the title of this book mentions orgasmic health it would be remiss of me, as a therapist, not to mention this important aspect of our life that can bring us so much joy, pleasure and satisfaction. There are so many benefits of having joyful sex. It releases endorphins: the feel-good factor, raises our self-esteem, heals our hearts, is a great form of exercise and helps us to feel loved, respected and valued. It is said that we can say many words to express how we feel about someone, and if we hugged them that would be far more potent and would convey far more than words ever could. With that in mind here are some of the strategies that help with having joyful and pleasurable sex. It is essential to make time so that it is not rushed or at the end of a very busy day. We are not at our best after a hard day's work and in Taoist terms it is said that the morning is the best time for sex, which they call Morning Prayer. It is believed that our energy is at its most potent and happy first thing in the morning.

All too often our days are busily mapped out with whatever work we do, our children's activities, taking care of elderly parents, escapism pastimes, which creates' tiredness and a lack of desire and excitement. Make time for this important activity. Try planning date nights, by that I mean take it in turns to decide what you'd like to do with your partner, for instance on a Friday night when there is no work the following day. Be creative, start with a light meal and then flirt with each other: the importance of anticipation and deliberate stimulation of desire cannot be stressed enough. Send erotic text messages to each other during the day, anticipating what you will be doing in the evening. Think about role-play and dressing up for each other. This adds excitement and can mean you have already excited each other and negotiated what you are going to do in your play time.

An interesting way of creating a mood for a sexy, sensual, tantalising, play time with your partner is to use a technique called Tantric sex: 'Awakening the senses with Tantra'. This takes a little bit of preparation, but is well worth the results. You can negotiate what foods you particularly like before the session starts. In Tantra the woman is pleasured first.

The man would ensure that his Goddess is wrapped in a sarong and is lying down on either a bed or on cushions. Once she is blindfolded, by taking away this sense it heightens all the others, and heightens the pleasure. There would be a tray with morsels of food on, which can include cubes of cheese, chocolate buttons, cherry tomatoes, nuts and seeds, and can involve all your favourite foods when planned in advance. There is another tray which has a variety of at least six essential oils. Then some musical instruments which could include rattles, a drum and a flute. A bag of different fabrics which might include lace, velvet, satin, seashells, pinecones, feathers and devices such as Angel fingers, which are copper rods that can be stroked over the body. The idea is that the man gives his Goddess scrumptious tastes, fabulous fragrances, beautiful music and sounds and strokes her skin with sensual materials. As she is blindfolded this has a tendency to heighten the senses. After drinking some water, it is then the man's turn. Your Goddess will pleasure you in much the same way which will help you to feel very intimate and loving.

The book *5 Primary Love Languages* by Jim Toole and Gary Chapman help us to understand in which language we, and our partner, experience being loved. The categories are physical touch, quality time, affirmations, gifts and presents, acts of service. So, imagine for a moment that what you give your partner from these categories is what you truly enjoy receiving. My primary love languages are physical touch and quality time, so I will give my partner lots of time, eye contact and listen carefully to what they are saying and will be hugging them and stroking them, as they are my primary love languages and are how I feel loved, respected and appreciated.

Problems may arise if my partner has different primary love languages, for instance if his primary love languages are affirmations and acts of service he will feel completely unloved by the way that I show my love to him in my two primary love languages. What he really needs is someone to tell him how wonderful, how handsome, how amazing he is and how well he has completed tasks. He would enjoy me helping in the tasks, or making his lunch box or making his favourite meal. Sometimes the reason that we don't feel loved and appreciated by our partner is simply that we speak a different language. I offer people an opportunity to explore their primary love languages with a questionnaire that has thirty paired statements which are read by you and you decide which one you would want to receive from your partner. At the end of the questionnaire we pull the totals of all the statements that you chose and this will give us which two primary love languages resonate with you most. This can make a significant difference to people once they have an understanding of their own primary love languages and their partners.

Choose your battles, choose to let go of the need to be right. This is so important, as sometimes we get so carried away with wanting to score points with our partner and prove that we are right, we end up being quite ruthless and hurting them, as well as ourselves, ultimately. So, decide if this is important enough to have a big row over, or is it something that you can just let go of. I'm not suggesting that we become submissive in our relationships. This is simply deciding to be loving rather than right.

This is something I've tried in the past and which has been delightful for my partner and I to experience, also it means making opportunities to 'flood your partner with affirmations'. You take it in turns to do this exercise and set a timer, for example in ten minutes you tell them all the wonderful, amazing, fantastic, qualities, attributes and gifts they possess until they are completely flooded with affirmations.

You then swap over and they do it for you. This is a wonderful opportunity to really affirm your partner and links in with another strategy which is catching your partner doing lovely things.

Instead of trying to find fault and noticing things that your partner does not do, try changing your perspective and look only for the good things that they do. Affirm them for what you've caught them doing. Tell them how much you appreciate what they did. This has a really positive effect on both the giver and the receiver and can encourage more laughter, more fun and more pleasure.

Another way of ensuring that you are literally on the same page as your partner is to find daily opportunities for dialoguing. This is an opportunity for checking where you are individually and as a couple. This needs to only take ten minutes. You basically set a question such as - What is my strongest feeling today? Then both parties write down their answers separately for ten minutes using "I" statements and talking about your feelings rather than just your thoughts. Start with an affirmation, for instance "My Darling..." and end it with lots of love. By checking in with each other daily means that misunderstandings don't develop into something more sinister and damaging. There is plenty of research that suggests that divorce is defined as a breakdown of a relationship that happens due to a lack of communication. It is rarely due to infidelity or any of the other so-called reasons why relationships end. According to Worldwide Marriage Encounter and Relate, the reason that relationships end is usually attributable to a breakdown in communication. Be honest, be truthful, be authentic. Claim your feelings and speak the truth. Always ensure that you've made your peace with each other before you go to sleep. Remember that you are always doing the best that you possibly can in any given circumstance and situation. If we could do any better, then we would already be doing it.

NOTE FROM THE AUTHOR

I trust that this little book of orgasmic health tips has been of value to you. I have truly enjoyed writing this book and if I can be of any service to you in the future please do not hesitate to contact me via email at annie@heavenscentbliss.co.uk or via telephone on 07869 123065.

With love, light and sparkling faery blessings Annie Day MSc. Cert Med Ed.

BIBLIOGRAPHY AND REFERENCES

ADAMS, J. (2007) *Researching Complementary and Alternative Medicine.* Oxon: Routledge.

ADAMO, J. and WHITNEY, C. (2016) *Eat Right 4 Your Type.* London: Pitman.

ALI, M. (2001) *The Integrated Health Bible: for optimum health and vitality.* London: Vermilion.

BALDWIN, D. S. and FOONG, T. (2013) Antidepressant drugs and sexual dysfunction. *The British Journal of Psychiatry, 202,* pp. 396-397.

BALON, R. and SEGRAVES, R. T. (2005) *Handbook of Sexual Dysfunction.* Boca Raton: Taylor and Francis.

BEDDOWS, K. (2012) Complementary therapies that help with overcoming infertility. *Natural Health Magazine (July),* pp. 4-6.

BOUL, L. and KERR, J. (2012) *DIY Sex and Relationship Therapy.* Oxford: How to Books.

CARLYLE, M. (2015) *Money magnet mind-set: Tools to keep*

you and your money on track. London: Hay House.

CHIA, M. and ABRAMS-ARAVA, D. (2001) *The Multi Orgasmic man: How any man can experience multiple orgasms and dramatically enhance his sexual relationship.* London: Thorson.

CHIA, M. and CARLTON, A. (2005) *The Multi Orgasmic woman: How any woman can experience ultimate pleasure and dramatically enhance her health and happiness.* California: Rodale Inc.

CHIA, M. (2006) *Teaching the multi orgasmic couple: working with sexual dysfunction and sexuality issues* [Lecture notes] Information for Taoist teachers / therapists. London. Ramada Hotel, Conference Room 7, 9 June 2006.

CLAYTON, P. (2001) *Health Defence.* Aylesbury: Accelerated Learning Publishing.

COLEMAN, S. (2002) *Complementary therapies that boost fertility.* California: Sage Publications.

CORMIER, Z. (2014) *Sex and Drugs and Rock N Roll: The Science of Hedonism the Hedonism of Science.* London: Profile Books.

CROCKER, P. (1999) *The healing herbs cook book.* Montréal: Canadian publishing.

DAVIS, P. (2011) *Subtle aromatherapy.* Essex: The CW Daniel Company Ltd.

DIABETES UK (2013) *Erectile Dysfunction Causes In men* [Online] Available from: http://www.diabetes.org-uk/Guide-to-diabetes/Living_with_diabetes.co.uk [Accessed 11/11/14]

DULLMAN, S., GROOT, J., KOSTER, D. and HEILGERS, P. (2010) Why Seek Complementary Medicine? An observational study in homeopathic, acupunctural and naturopathic medical practices. *Journal of Complementary and Integrative Medicine, 1,* pp. 7-9.

DONALDSON, J. (2008) *The psychological aspects of essential oils.* Bristol: Self-publish.

EDEN, D. (2005) *Energy Medicine: Using your bodies' energies to balance and heal.* Somerset: The Bath Press.

EMOTO, M. (2005) *The Hidden Messages in Water.* Oregon: Beyond Words Publishing.

ERNST, E. (2007) Evaluation of complementary and alternative medicine. *Journal for Quality in Health Care [Online] 101 (5)* Available from: http://www.sciencedirect.com/science/article/pii/s143176210 7001236 [Accessed 20/1/15]

ERNST, E., POSADZKI, P. and LEE, M. (2011)

Complementary and alternative medicine (CAM) for sexual dysfunction and erectile dysfunction in older men and women: an overview of systematic reviews. *Maturitas, 70,* pp. 37-41.

FEDERATION of HOLISTIC THERAPISTS (2015) *Handbook for Holistic Therapists.* Cardiff: FHT.

FRENKEL, M. and BORKAN, J. (2003) An Approach for integrating complementary – alternative medicine into primary care. *Journal of Family Practitioners, 20,* pp. 324–332.

FRENKEL, M., ARYE, E., CARLSON, C. and SIERPINA, V. (2008) Integrating Complementary and Alternative Medicine into Conventional Primary Care: The Patient Perspective. *Journal of Science and Healing, 4 (3),* pp.178–186.

GERBER, R. (2002) *Vibrational medicine in the 21st century: a complete guide to energy healing and spiritual transformation.* New York: William Morrow and Company.

GREAT BRITAIN, HOUSE of LORDS REPORT on COMPLEMENTARY and ALTERNATIVE MEDICINE (CAM) [2000] [Online] Chapter 2 Available from: http://www.publications.parliament.uk/pa/ld199900/ldscetech /123/12301.htm [Accessed 10/3/15]

HALL, K. and GRAHAM, C. (2012) *The Cultural Context of*

Sexual Pleasure and Problems: Psychotherapy with Diverse Clients. London: Routledge.

Holford, P. (2009) *The Optimum Nutrition Bible.* London: Piatkus.

KEMP, A. (2006) *Quantum K: Returning to our original blueprint.* Bristol: Andrew J. Kemp.

LEIBLUM, S. (2007). *Principles and Practice of Sex Therapy,* 4th Ed. New York: Guilford.

LITTLE, C. (2009) Simply because it works better. Exploring motives for the use of medical herbalism in contemporary UK health care. *Journal of Complementary therapy medicine 17 (6),* pp. 300–308.

LITTLE, C. (2013) Integrative health care: implications for nursing practice and education. *British Journal of Nursing 22 (20),* pp. 773-777.

LITVINOFF, S. (2003) *Sex in Loving Relationships: The Relate Guide.* London: Vermillion.

NEALS YARD (2013) *Healing Foods.* London: Dorling Kindersley.

O'CONNOR, D. (1997) *How to make love to the same person for the rest of your life: and still love it!* London: Virgin Books.

ONG, V. (2014) *Eurycoma Longifolia - Malaysian Ginseng: The Safe and Effective Sexual Health Enhancing Herb.* The Magazine of Chinese Medicine (March), pp. 12-14.

PATTERSON, C. (2001) Primary Health Care transformed: complementary and orthodox medicine complementing each other. *Journal of Complementary Therapies and Medicine, 8,* pp. 47–49.

PEASE, B. (2003) *Why men lie and women cry.* London: Orion.

PORTERBROOK NHS SEX CLINIC, SHEFFIELD (2012) Internal leaflets and Hand-outs for Sex Therapists on Sexual health and Sexuality Issues (Sept- Jan).

ROBINSON, P. (2010) *Impotency causes and natural remedies.* Sexual Health Magazine (November), pp. 5-8.

READER'S DIGEST (2001) *Foods that harm foods that heal.* London: Readers Digest.

SCHNARCH, D. (2013) *Resurrecting Sex: Solving Problems and Revolutionizing Your Relationship.* California: Harper Collins.

SWEETSER, W. (2010) *Smoothie Heaven.* London: Apple Press.

WICKS, J. (2016) *Lean in 15 - the shape plan.* London:

Bluebird.

WILSON, S. (2016) *I quit sugar: Simplicious.* London: McMillan.

WONG, J. (2009) *Grow your own drugs.* London: Harper-Collins.

ZEILINSKI, R. (2013) Assessment of Women's Sexual health using a Holistic patient centred approach. *Journal of Midwifery and Women's Health, 58 (3),* pp. 321-327.